Innovative Tools for Health Education

Making Inexpensive Props, Visuals, and Manipulatives

Marilyn Grechus, PhD

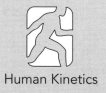

Human Kinetics

Library of Congress Cataloging-in-Publication Data

Grechus, Marilyn, 1948-
Innovative tools for health education : making inexpensive props, visuals, and manipulatives / Marilyn Grechus.
    p. cm.
ISBN-13: 978-0-7360-8985-2 (soft cover)
ISBN-10: 0-7360-8985-3 (soft cover)
    1. Health education--Audio-visual aids. 2. Teaching--Aids and devices--Design and construction. I. Title.
    RA440.55.G74 2010
    613.071--dc22

                                            2009039157

ISBN-10: 0-7360-8985-3 (print)
ISBN-13: 978-0-7360-8985-2 (print)

Copyright © 2010 by Marilyn Grechus

Acquisitions Editor: Sarajane Quinn; **Managing Editor:** Bethany J. Bentley; **Assistant Editors:** Derek Campbell and Elizabeth Evans; **Copyeditor:** Jan Feeney; **Graphic Designer:** Nancy Rasmus; **Graphic Artist:** Dawn Sills; **Cover Designer:** Keith Blomberg; **Photographer (cover):** Courtesy of Marilyn Grechus; **Photographs (interior):** Courtesy of Marilyn Grechus; **Photo Production Manager:** Jason Allen; **Art Manager:** Kelly Hendren; **Associate Art Manager:** Alan L. Wilborn; **Illustrator:** Mike Meyer; **Printer:** Versa Press

Printed in the United States of America   10 9 8 7 6 5 4 3 2 1

The paper in this book is certified under a sustainable forestry program.

Human Kinetics
Web site: www.HumanKinetics.com

United States: Human Kinetics
P.O. Box 5076
Champaign, IL 61825-5076
800-747-4457
e-mail: humank@hkusa.com

Canada: Human Kinetics
475 Devonshire Road Unit 100
Windsor, ON N8Y 2L5
800-465-7301 (in Canada only)
e-mail: info@hkcanada.com

Europe: Human Kinetics
107 Bradford Road
Stanningley
Leeds LS28 6AT, United Kingdom
+44 (0) 113 255 5665
e-mail: hk@hkeurope.com

Australia: Human Kinetics
57A Price Avenue
Lower Mitcham, South Australia 5062
08 8372 0999
e-mail: info@hkaustralia.com

New Zealand: Human Kinetics
PO Box 80
Torrens Park, SA, 5062
0800 222 062
e-mail: info@hknewzealand.com

E5033

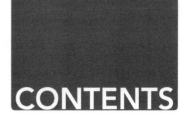

CONTENTS

We've all heard these deflating words: "Sorry. We can't afford that right now." Yet school districts expect teachers to provide a top-notch education to all students. Quite a dilemma—and one that will continue in most schools. There is never enough money, especially for the health and physical education curriculum. But such predicaments often present an opportunity for creativity. This is especially true when creating teaching materials for the health classroom. A little thought and some guidance from this book will provide the teaching tools you need in order to make an impact on students. What's more, these teaching materials will fit into the budget of almost any school district.

Innovative Tools for Health Education is a guide for all teachers who are short on funds for teaching props for health lessons, but feeling like their students are the ones who are short-changed when the props are not available. Whether you teach health classes in elementary school or high school, this book will take you step by step through the process of using everyday materials and turning them into props that can enhance every student's health lessons. There are 28 projects plus several ideas for reusing and purchasing inexpensive substitutes for more expensive catalog items. The simple instructions are accompanied by photographs of materials and the steps involved in assembly. There is also a statement or two of how the props can be incorporated into lessons.

These ideas have come from years of creating materials to be used for demonstrating teaching methods in workshops and conferences I have presented across the United States. Health teachers, science teachers, and school nurses have all had positive comments about how useful a book like this would be since most schools are short on resources.

These ideas will give teachers a new perspective on how to look at ordinary objects lying around the house. With a little time and energy, items that you'd pay a lot of money for in the catalogs can be made for pennies. You will have the pleasure of knowing that students are gaining new insights into their health because of the teaching props available to them. Your students will certainly be healthier for it.

The most unique thing about this book is that any teacher will find ideas that could enhance their teaching. The ideas encompassed in the book are specifically for teaching health, but many of them could supplement other lessons as well. For example, the puppets made from stuffed animals could easily be used in language arts. The easel could be used to display any small project.

Teachers are generally creative people, but they sometimes need some inspiration to get started. Hopefully, the ideas in this book will spark some enthusiasm for being resourceful and help teachers emerge with a sense of accomplishment and the knowledge that their students will be more attentive to their health lessons. With a little time, effort, and just a little cash, any teacher can enhance their inventory of teaching aids. Give it a try! What is there to lose?

Acknowledgments

My special thanks go to Dr. Sheri Beeler at Missouri Southern University, Julie Leukenhoff at Blair Oaks High School, and Marla Drewel-Lynch for their ideas. These educators care about their students and understand how their jobs are limited by their schools' budgets. They have used many of these ideas in their own teaching and have shared with me what they have used.

I also want to thank my brother, Lee Hancock, who took the time to help me photograph the items. Without his help and support, this book would still be on my back burner!

ACTIVITIES

Portable First Aid Kit

Elementary classroom teachers (and any other adults who take students out of the school building) need a way to carry first aid supplies with them every time they leave their classrooms. This kit is simple enough that every teacher should have her own to hang right inside the door so it can be grabbed on the way out.

Materials

- Small, inexpensive travel pack
- First aid supplies (determined by district policies or school nurse):
  - Plastic or vinyl gloves
  - 2-inch (5 cm) athletic tape
  - Rolled gauze
  - 2-by-2-inch gauze pads
  - Plastic adhesive bandages (variety of sizes)
  - Antibiotic ointment
  - Cleansing towelettes
  - Alcohol wipes
  - Tweezers
  - Cold pack
  - Elastic bandage
  - Tylenol
  - Hard candy or sugar packets

Instructions for Assembling

1. Collect materials.
2. Assemble basic first aid supplies into travel pack and place in a convenient spot near the exit (figure 1.1).

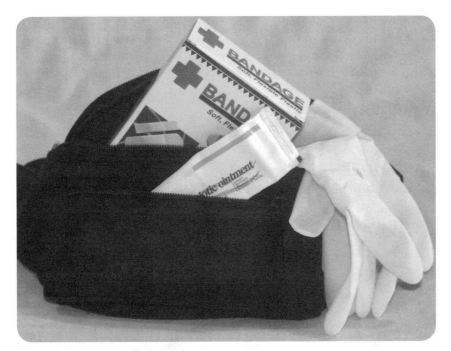

Figure 1.1 Travel pack supplies.

To Use

Place by door to have available every time you leave the classroom. Use it as a teaching aid to show students how to create their own first aid kits to have at home.

Stethoscope

Children love to use stethoscopes for listening to their—or others'—hearts. Although store-bought stethoscopes are not very expensive, the homemade versions can be much more appealing. And, if the materials are donated, children can take the stethoscopes home with them!

Materials (Figure 2.1)

- Small funnel (approximately 2 inches in diameter and 2 inches long)
- T coupling (found in the plumbing department or automotive department of a hardware store)
- Hollow rubber or plastic tubing (such as exercise tubing, surgical tubing, or plastic jump rope)

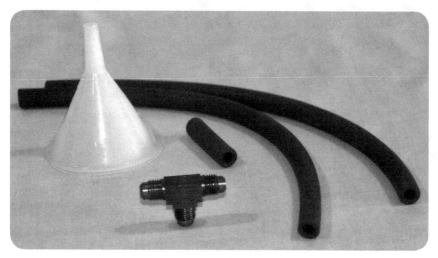

Figure 2.1   Materials for stethoscope.

Instructions for Assembling

1. Cut tubing into three pieces. Two pieces are approximately 12 inches (30 cm) long and one piece is 3 inches (8 cm) long (figure 2.1).
2. Attach the funnel to one end of the 3-inch piece of tubing (figure 2.2).
3. Attach the bottom end of the T coupling to the other end of the 3-inch piece of tubing (figure 2.2).
4. Attach the long pieces of tubing to either side of the top piece of the T coupling (figure 2.2).
5. Work pieces of tubing snugly onto coupling and funnel so it doesn't come apart easily.

If you wish to disassemble and keep, store in zipped plastic bags.

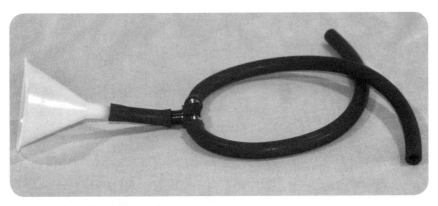

Figure 2.2   Assembled stethoscope.

To Use

The long pieces of tubing go into the ears. The funnel is held against the chest to pick up the sound of the beating heart. Use it when teaching students about increased heart rate caused by exercise or activity.

If more than one student uses the same stethoscope, you can disinfect with alcohol wipes between uses.

Puppets

All children love puppets! Most children will interact with a puppet in ways they won't with an adult. Unfortunately, puppets are not always available in the characters you want or need. A simple solution is to transform an appropriate stuffed animal into a puppet.

Materials

- Stuffed animals (almost any size will work—larger animals will make hand puppets, and smaller can be finger puppets); don't forget to look in the pet department, too!
- Craft knife (box cutter type) or seam ripper (sewing tool)
- Old mitten or glove
- Scraps of material for finger puppets
- Hot-glue gun

Instructions for Assembling

Larger Stuffed Animal

1. Carefully cut open a part of the seam to the body of the animal (where you want to be able to insert your hand).
2. Remove enough of the stuffing so that a hand can be inserted.
3. Glue (using a hot-glue gun) or stitch a mitten or glove into the opening. This lets the user insert a hand without being concerned about the stuffing (figure 3.1). (This is especially important if children use the puppet.)

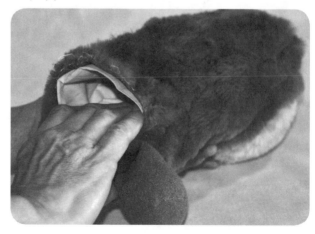

Figure 3.1 Ensure the opening is large enough for your hand to fit inside.

Small Stuffed Animals

1. You can follow the instructions for the larger stuffed animal if appropriate, or follow the instructions in this section.

2. Glue both ends of a strip of cloth (approximately 1 by 3 inches, or 2.5 by 8 cm) to the back of the animal, allowing room for a finger to slide under it so you can animate the puppet (figures 3.2 and 3.3).

3. If you can't find a strip of cloth in the color you want (to match the animal), you can use a permanent marker to color the cloth (figure 3.3).

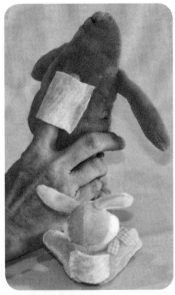

Figure 3.2 Use a cloth strip on the outside for smaller animals.

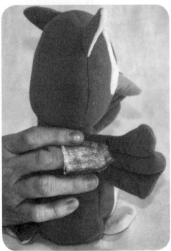

Figure 3.3 Color the cloth to match the animal, if desired.

To Use

Use as you would any puppet to engage your students in conversations or in learning appropriate healthy behaviors. Use in role-plays or skits or as a "guest" lecturer.

Beanbags

Students enjoy activities with tactile manipulatives. These can be used in a variety of activities or games.

Materials

- Heavy plastic (recycle an old inflatable toy such as a child's bop bag that leaks)
- Scissors
- Permanent markers in various colors
- Polyurethane spray paint
- Baby powder
- Sewing machine (or needle and thread)
- Rice or beans

Instructions for Assembling

1. Cut two circles (3.5 to 4 inches in diameter, or 9 to 10 cm) for each beanbag. (Trace around a small dish; figure 4.1).
2. Using the permanent markers, draw a fruit or vegetable on one side. The name of the fruit or vegetable can be written on the back side (figure 4.2).

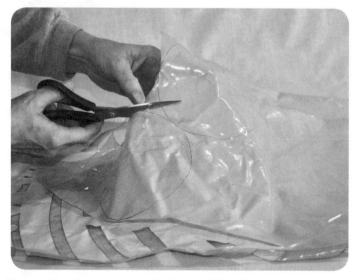

Figure 4.1 Cut out two circles for each beanbag.

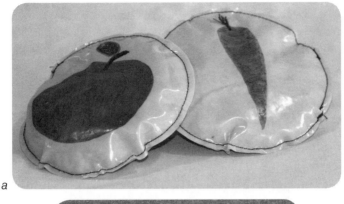

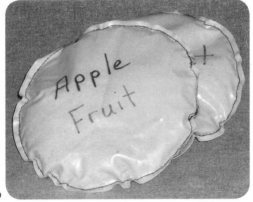

Figure 4.2 *(a)* Use permanent markers to draw a vegetable or fruit on one side. *(b)* On the back side, write the name of the fruit or vegetable.

3. After the marker dries, spray very lightly with the polyurethane paint and let dry completely. Once it is dry, dust lightly with baby powder and rub it in. Wipe off excess. (This keeps the marker or paint from being sticky.)

4. Sew around the edge, leaving an opening for inserting the filling.

5. Fill with rice or small beans.

6. Sew up opening.

To Use

Create a game, such as toss to a teammate who then has to name the fruit or vegetable shown on the beanbag. As a variation, the teammate could name the food group or spell the name.

Health Balls

Some students are very resistant to joining an activity. They prefer to sit and watch or totally disengage themselves from the class. You can draw students back in by including them in the tossing and catching of the balls.

Materials

- Blown-up beach ball or other inexpensive plastic ball
- Permanent markers
- Polyurethane spray paint

Instructions for Assembling

1. Select topic for the activity (such as substance use and abuse, mental health, nutrition).
2. Blow up ball if needed.
3. Using permanent markers, write statements or questions all over the ball. You can also use pictures to represent statements (figure 5.1). For example, stars could represent this statement: "I am good at ___." Hearts could mean "I like ___." To add texture and interest, you can use foam stickers in a variety of shapes.
4. Let marker dry completely.
5. Spray lightly with polyurethane paint. Allow to dry completely. If it's sticky, dust very lightly with baby powder.

To Use

Put students into groups of five to seven. A student will toss the ball to a peer in the group. The statement or question closest to where the right thumb (or other preselected digit) lands is what the student will do or answer. That student then tosses the ball to someone else. Be sure to explain to groups that everyone should be included. This can be used as an icebreaker or a review of information on the specific topic.

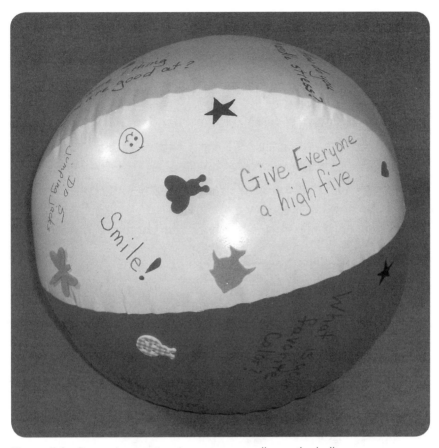

Figure 5.1   Draw pictures or write statements all over the ball.

Stress Balls

Stress balls are generally recognized as compact foam shapes that can be squeezed to help alleviate stress. This concept is beneficial for students who are often dealing with multiple stressors. If students are allowed to create their own stress balls, it can give them a sense of empowerment that will benefit them in other areas of their lives.

Materials (Figure 6.1)

- Heavy balloons (at least 9 inches), two for each stress ball
- Fillers (flour, salt, sand, rice, small beans, or any combination)
- Permanent markers (if you want to decorate the balls)
- Baby powder (if you decorate the balls)
- Funnel or 2-liter or smaller plastic drink bottle to make a funnel

Instructions for Assembling

1. To make a funnel, cut off the open end of a plastic drink bottle (about 3 inches, or 8 cm, down the bottle).
2. Roll one balloon lengthwise into a small roll that can then be inserted into a second balloon. This will give a double thickness to the ball (figure 6.2).
3. Insert funnel spout (the screw-top portion of the bottle) into the neck of the double balloon.

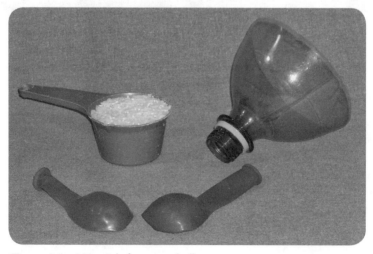

Figure 6.1   Materials for stress ball.

Innovative Tools for Health Education

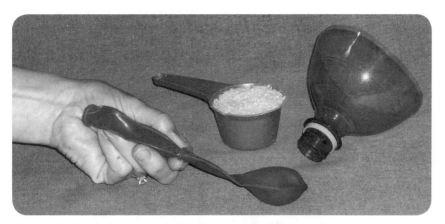

Figure 6.2 One balloon inserted into a second balloon.

4. Fill with the filler material of your choice until the balloon is tightly filled (figure 6.3).

5. Remove funnel and tie the neck of the balloons into a knot to keep filler inside.

6. Decorate with permanent markers if desired. Let it dry completely before dusting lightly with baby powder.

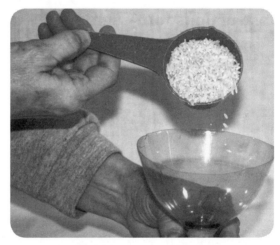

Figure 6.3 Use the funnel to fill up the balloon.

To Use

Squeeze for stress reduction. Some students might use the ball as a manipulative to squeeze as they are studying or practicing spelling words.

Germs Under the Black Light

Students are often told to wash their hands to get rid of germs. But, because germs cannot be seen, this is a difficult concept for most children to comprehend. If you allow students to see how germs are on the hands and are spread, students are more likely to understand the importance of proper hand washing for the prevention of illness.

Materials

- Liquid laundry detergent (preferably for infants to reduce the chance of allergies)
- Small bottle with lid for the liquid
- Powdered presoak or powdered bleach
- Small container with lid for powder

Instructions for Assembling

1. Put the liquid laundry detergent in a small bottle (figure 7.1).
2. Powder can be ground into a finer powder in a blender, if desired.
3. Put powder in a container that will be easier to handle.

To Use

Students will put a small amount of the liquid soap on their hands and rub it in as if it were hand lotion. Look at hands under a black light. Their hands will glow. Then have students wash their hands. The soap washes off easily, but the whiteners in the detergent don't, so the hands still glow under the black light. Hands must be scrubbed with soap and water to wash off the whiteners.

To show how germs spread, place some powder on the students' hands and let them touch things around them. The places where the powder has been deposited will glow under the black light. You can also put the powder on an object (such as a stuffed animal) and pass the object around to see if the "germ" powder is being passed to others who handle the object. Check hands under the black light.

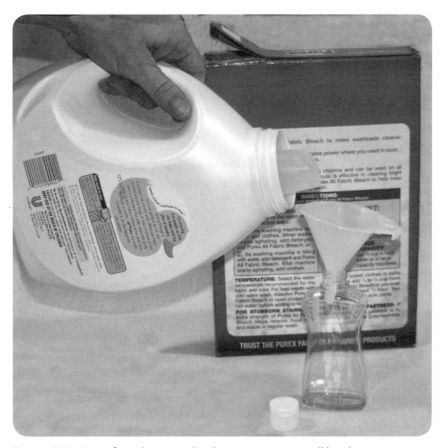

Figure 7.1 Use a funnel to pour the detergent into a small bottle.

Alcohol Goggles

The effects of alcohol are difficult to replicate. These goggles simulate the visual impairment that accompanies drinking alcohol. Students may experience feelings such as nausea and disorientation. To show the effects of alcohol impairment on physical skills, you can have students do coordination activities while wearing the goggles.

Materials (Figure 8.1)

Option A
Gel relaxation eye mask (The one I used has a 'citrus veins' motif over the eyes. As you look through the gel and lines, your vision is impaired.)

Option B
- Snack-size plastic zip bags
- Duct tape (or similar heavy tape)
- Clear hair gel
- Clear or colored safety goggles or large sunglasses

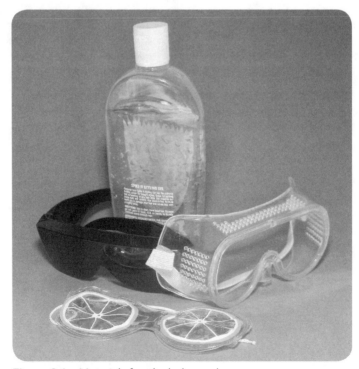

Figure 8.1 Materials for alcohol goggles.

Instructions for Assembling

Option A
Use the eye mask just as it is or tape it to a pair of safety goggles.

Option B
1. Put enough clear hair gel into a snack-size plastic zip bag so that you fill it yet allow it to remain flat. Close securely.
2. Use duct tape to reinforce the closed side so it does not leak. If you have narrow tape, you could also reinforce the sides and bottom seams of the bag.
3. Tape the bag to the front of the goggles to create the simulation of impaired vision. Store flat (lay the bag flat to keep the gel spread out evenly in the bag).

To Use

Use as you would the ready-made goggles. Have students try walking a line, tossing a ball to a friend, screwing nuts onto bolts, and so on while wearing the goggles. The distortion makes everyday activities much more challenging.

DUI Game Kit

This game is used in conjunction with the alcohol goggles. The premise of the game is to put on the goggles, throw a Velcro ball at a large targeted area, and suffer the consequences of your simulated drinking and driving.

Materials

- Flannel-backed plastic tablecloth (52 inches, or about 130 cm, square or small oblong)
- Permanent markers
- Velcro-covered plastic ball (these come with inexpensive dart games)

Instructions for Assembling

1. Use markers to section off portions on the flannel (cloth) side of the tablecloth. (You can refer to a picture in a catalog if you need specific ideas.)
2. Write scenarios in sections. Here are examples: Ran into a tree and ended up in a wheelchair. Hit another car and killed a family. Got home safely (figure 9.1).
3. Hang so that it is not directly against a wall because the ball will bounce off of the hard surface of the wall. You can hang a rope between two shelving units or across a wide doorway.
4. Use clothespins to secure the top of the tablecloth to the rope.

To Use

Wearing the alcohol goggles, a student throws the Velcro-covered ball at the scenario-covered tablecloth. Students will have to "pay" for their impaired vision with the consequence their ball lands on. This can be a great discussion starter on actions having consequences and taking responsibility for actions.

Variation

This type of game board can be made for any topic or type of game.

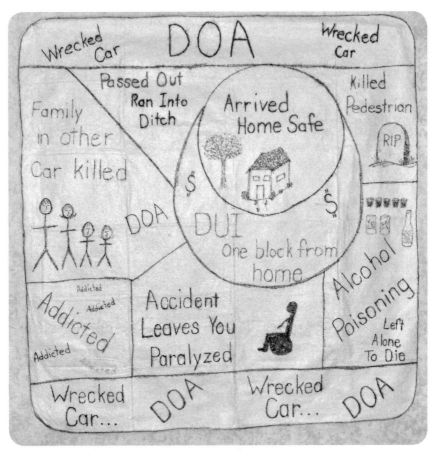

Figure 9.1   Sample scenarios for DUI game kit.

Bottles With Impact

Visuals are very important in helping to make a point with young people. Since there is no way to show someone just how drugs can hurt an unborn child, you can—at the very least—make students stop and think about how their actions affect the children they (or a friend) will one day have.

Materials (Figure 10.1)

- Clear plastic baby bottles (small sizes work great)
- Items to put inside, such as beer bottle caps, cigarette butts, and various pills; alternative items could be candy, chips, and cookies (figure 10.2)

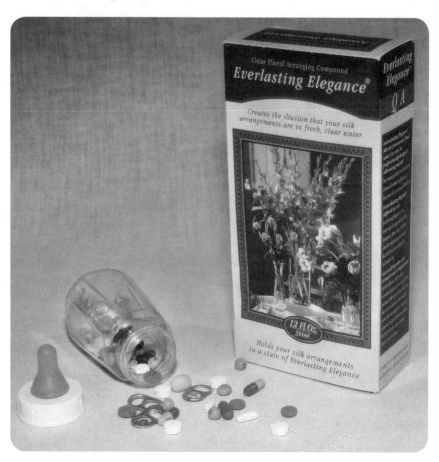

Figure 10.1 Materials for bottles with impact.

Innovative Tools for Health Education

- Acrylic resin (Everlasting Elegance and Quick Water are available at craft stores; one package, though not cheap, will make two 4-ounce bottles)
- Old plastic bowl or container to mix it in
- Plastic spoon or Popsicle stick for stirring the resin
- Small card (1 by 2 inches, or 2.5 by 5 cm) and narrow ribbon (12 inches, or 30 cm, long) to tie the card onto the finished bottle

Instructions for Assembling

1. Assemble all materials on a newspaper-covered table.
2. Follow the instructions for mixing the acrylic resin in your old plastic bowl with the plastic spoon or stick.
3. As you pour the resin into the bottles, add the drug-related items and pills. Fill resin up to where the nipple screws onto the bottle.
4. Do not disturb the bottle as you allow the resin to harden completely.
5. Screw the nipple on.
6. Write on the card any message you want, such as "Would you feed this to *your* baby?"
7. Punch a hole in the card if you want to use a piece of narrow ribbon to tie it around the neck of the bottle.

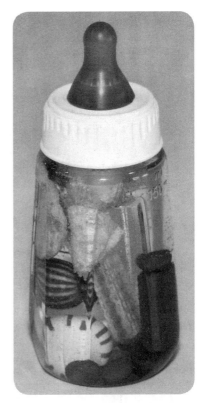

Figure 10.2 Bottle filled with candy.

To Use

Discuss how everything that goes into the pregnant (or nursing) woman's body also goes into the baby. And the baby doesn't have a choice.

Breathless Cigarettes

People who smoke are deprived of adequate oxygen. Breathing through these "cigarettes" simulates how it feels to be deprived of air, which is what happens when a person becomes a smoker.

Materials

- Drinking straws that are approximately the same diameter as a cigarette (best if either clear or white)
- Cotton (2 or 3 cotton balls, depending on how many cigarettes you are making)
- Tweezers
- Scissors
- Optional: hinged metal cigarette container or empty cigarette pack

Instructions for Assembling

1. Cut the straws into lengths to represent cigarettes. (If you will use a cigarette container to store them, cut to fit the container; figure 11.1).
2. Use tweezers to poke cotton loosely into the straws.
3. Don't pack the cigarettes too tightly because they will be too difficult to breathe through.

Leave half an inch or so of space on each end so that when students put the cigarettes into their mouths, they won't get the cotton into their mouths.

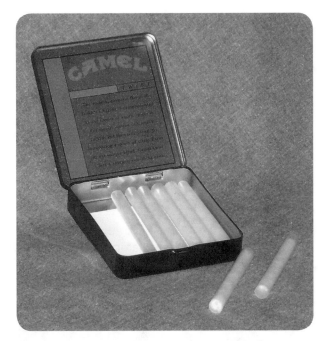

Figure 11.1 Straws cut to represent cigarettes.

To Use

Students can put these cigarettes into their mouths and gently inhale and exhale through them to represent how difficult it is for smokers to catch their breath. This type of simulation is a great discussion starter for athletes, as well as other students, on the hazards of smoking.

Breathless Cigarettes 23

Smokeless Tobacco Can

The giant can opens to a pair of giant dice containing pictures of the consequences of using smokeless tobacco. It can be used just as a display, or students can roll the dice for a more personal view of what can happen to *them*.

Materials

- Round papier-mâché box, any size (from a craft store; figure 12.1)
- Spray paint (colors to match the brand of smokeless tobacco most popular in your community)
- Permanent markers
- Plain paper (any type, any color)
- Pictures of problems caused by smokeless tobacco (available from American Cancer Society pamphlets or the Internet)
- Giant dice (refer to page 56 for instructions on making them)
- Hot-glue gun or white glue

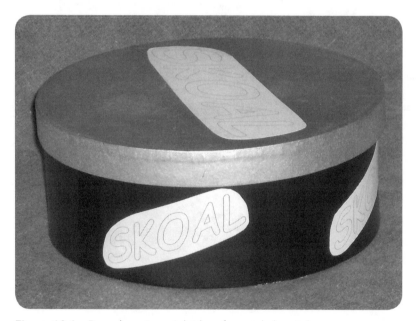

Figure 12.1   Round papier-mâché box for smokeless tobacco can.

Instructions for Assembling

1. Spray-paint the box inside and out to resemble a real smokeless tobacco can. Decorate it with the permanent markers as much as you want.

2. Inside the box lid and bottom of the box you can add circles of paper with messages written on them, such as "How lucky do you feel?" "Roll the die to see what can happen if *you* use" (figure 12.2).

3. Make dice.

4. Cut pictures of problems caused by smokeless tobacco to fit on the sides of the die.

5. Glue the pictures to the sides of the die. (White glue if you use paper dice, hot-glue gun if you use sponge dice; figure 12.2).

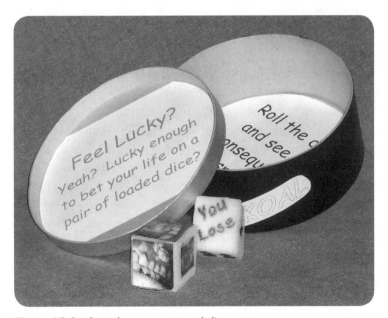

Figure 12.2 Sample messages and dice.

To Use

Set box up as a display for a discussion starter, or create a game allowing students to roll the dice inside the box to see the consequences of their use of smokeless tobacco.

Homemade Phlegm

Young people are always fascinated by bodily functions, but when you show them the amount of phlegm a person with emphysema coughs up in a day or two, it's just plain *disgusting!*

Materials (Figure 13.1)

- 2 cups of water
- 1 packet of plain gelatin
- 2 cups of sugar
- 4 rennet tablets (used in making homemade ice cream)
- Quart jar with lid (or something comparable, preferably in plastic rather than glass)
- Material for making label for jar (adhesive-backed printer paper works great; contact paper can secure plain paper labels)

Instructions for Assembling

1. Bring water to a boil in a medium saucepan.
2. Stir in remaining ingredients until everything is dissolved. Let boil a couple of minutes.
3. Allow mixture to cool. Put it in the refrigerator to speed the process.
4. Pour into jar and seal tightly. (It may not seem very gelatinous at first, but it sets after a little time in the refrigerator.) It can also be processed in a hot-water canner if put into a glass jar.
5. Print up a sign to put on the jar: "This represents the amount of phlegm a person with emphysema usually coughs up in a day or two."
6. If not canned, it can be stored in the refrigerator indefinitely.

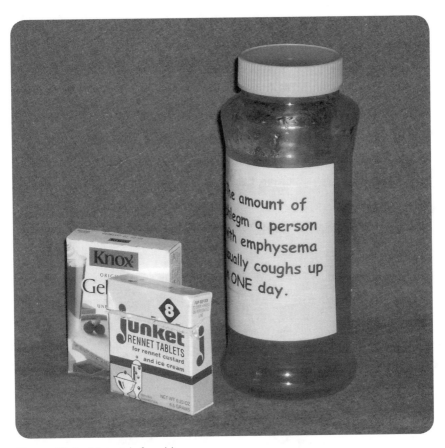

Figure 13.1 Materials for phlegm.

To Use

Use as a demonstration model in a tobacco unit. Pass it around and let the students handle it.

Tobacco Tar

This model demonstrates the amount of tar that accumulates in the lungs of a pack-a-day smoker in a few months' time.

Materials

- Quart jar (preferably plastic; figure 14.1 shows a plastic 24-ounce soda bottle)
- Molasses (approximately 20 ounces, or about 600 ml)
- Material for making sign for jar
- Optional: 6 to 8 cigarette butts

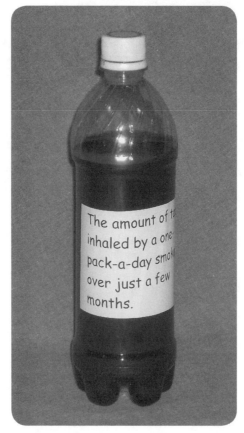

The amount of ta[r] inhaled by a one-pack-a-day smok[er] over just a few months.

Figure 14.1 Sample bottle of tar.

Instructions for Assembling

1. Pour molasses into jar.
2. Add cigarette butts if desired.
3. Seal tightly.
4. Add sign: "This is the amount of tar that accumulates in a pack-a-day smoker's lungs in just a few months" (figure 14.1).

To Use

Use this as a demonstration of the amount of tar that collects in the lungs as a person continues to smoke. Pass the jar around and let students see how this gooey liquid lines the inside of the jar. Relate this to what it does in a person's lungs.

Stinky Beanbag

People who smoke usually do not realize just how disgusting their clothes and breath smell. This model will make people more aware of how repulsive stale tobacco smells.

Materials

- Scraps of cloth (1 porous and 1 tightly woven)
- Scissors
- Cloth adhesive or sewing machine
- Permanent markers for decorating (if desired)
- Cigarette butts
- Rice for stuffing
- Hook-and-loop tape for closure
- Closed container or plastic zip bag for storage

Instructions for Assembling

1. Cut out a small rectangle or other shape from a double layer of porous cloth.
2. Hot-glue the layers together, leaving an opening to stuff with cigarette butts (figure 15.1). After it is filled, glue the last part closed.

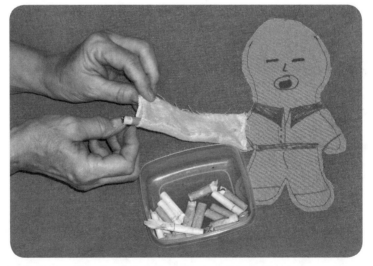

Figure 15.1   Glue the cloth layers together, then stuff with cigarette butts.

Innovative Tools for Health Education

3. Cut out the shape for a beanbag from a double layer of tightly woven cloth.

4. Decorate one or both sides of the beanbag (if desired).

5. Use adhesive or sew the two pieces together, leaving an opening for stuffing. Sew hook-and-loop tape into the opening for changing the smelly cigarette-butt-filled bag.

6. Fill beanbag loosely with rice and include the smelly cigarette-butt-filled bag (figure 15.2).

7. Store in a closed container or plastic zip bag.

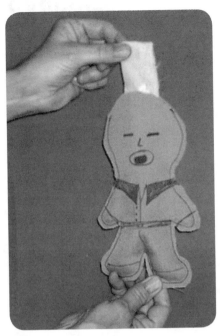

Figure 15.2 Put the cigarette-filled bag into the beanbag, along with the rice.

To Use

Students can smell the most disgusting smell known to humans. It far exceeds smelly feet!

Variation

You can make several of the cigarette-butt bags at one time so that you're ready to make refills as the odor dissipates. Don't fill them until ready to use.

Clogged Arteries

This model demonstrates how plaque (fatty acids) builds up in your blood vessels. The progression shows the advancing stages.

Materials

- Sturdy paper towel tubes
- Sharp knife or saw to cut the tubes
- Spray paint (dark red to represent the blood vessels)
- Clay that will harden (see page 64 for an easy recipe for home-made clay)
- Piece of heavy corrugated cardboard 6 by 12 inches (size can vary according to any extras you want to put on your display; cardboard can be painted or covered with paper or contact paper)
- Heavy glue (tacky craft glue)

Instructions for Assembling

1. Cut paper towel tubes into approximately 2-inch (5 cm) lengths. You need five small pieces.
2. Spray-paint the cut tubes inside and out. Allow to dry completely.
3. Leave one tube empty. Add clay to the insides in increasing amounts until the fifth one is almost totally blocked. (Keep the clay inside the tubes so that the tubes will sit flat.) Allow clay to dry.
4. Prepare the cardboard base. It could be spray-painted or covered with paper or contact paper.
5. Arrange the small tubes so the progression of fill goes from left to right (figure 16.1).
6. Use a heavy glue to secure the tubes in place. (Hot glue will not stick to contact paper.)
7. You can add small cards that describe what is happening.
8. For an easel to hold the model, recycle the stand from a day-by-day calendar (figure 16.2).

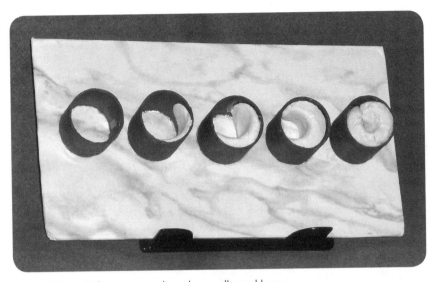

Figure 16.1 Tubes arranged on the cardboard base.

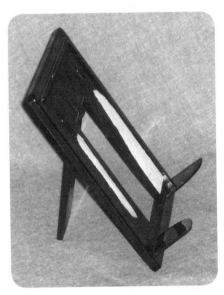

To Use

Students can examine the model as a discussion is held on how the opening of the blood vessel shrinks as the fat accumulates. This accumulation can be caused by a diet high in saturated fat and trans fat.

Figure 16.2 Recycled stand from a day-by-day calendar.

Components of Blood

Students sometimes have a difficult time visualizing what the inside of the body looks like. This model can be used to illustrate what blood is composed of.

Materials

- Clear tubular plastic bottle approximately 6 inches (15 cm) long and 1.5 inches (4 cm) in diameter (available in craft stores, or use a small lotion or shampoo bottle)
- Sharp craft knife
- 5 or 6 red flattened glass balls approximately a half-inch in diameter (like the ones used in fish tanks or flower or candle arrangements)
- 3 or 4 star-shaped beads approximately 3/8 inch in diameter
- 3 or 4 white marbles
- Hot-glue gun
- Cardboard for display board approximately 8 by 8 inches (20 cm square)
- Paper for covering the display board and for making signs

Instructions for Assembling

1. Clean bottle if it's recycled.
2. Cut a rectangle out of the side of the bottle about 1 inch (2.5 cm) wide, stopping approximately 1/2 inch (1 cm) from each end. Do not throw cutout piece away.
3. Use hot-glue gun to glue in the components of blood (red glass balls, beads, and marbles; refer to pictures in the catalogs if you want). Save one of each component for the next step.
4. Make small cards describing what each blood component does.
5. Take the piece removed from the bottle and cut off three pieces 1/2 inch wide.
6. Glue a blood component onto the raised side of each small piece.
7. Glue the corresponding component to the card.
8. Cover the display board.
9. Assemble your display (figure 17.1).

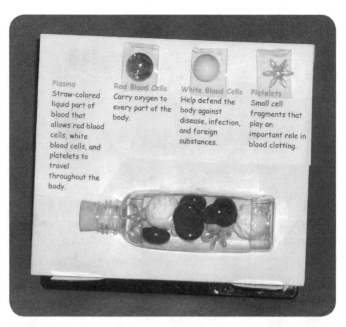

Figure 17.1 Assembled blood component board.

To Use

As students are studying the circulatory system, you can use this as a visual aid of what blood looks like.

Variation

You can use the stand from a day-by-day calendar for an easel (figure 17.2).

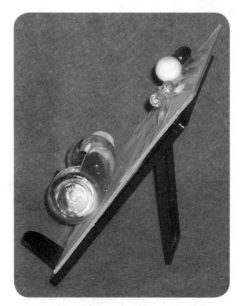

Figure 17.2 Reused day-by-day calendar.

Organ Vest

Students can gain a better understanding of what the inside of the body looks like by placing the organs in the correct spots.

Materials

- Old sweatshirt that has plenty of fleece on the inside
- Scissors
- Permanent markers
- Hook-and-loop tape

Instructions for Assembling

1. Cut neck binding and waistband from the sweatshirt. Cut sleeves from sweatshirt. Turn it inside out (figure 18.1).
2. Use the fabric from the sleeves to cut out the organs. (See appendix for patterns to enlarge.) Remember to cut the organs

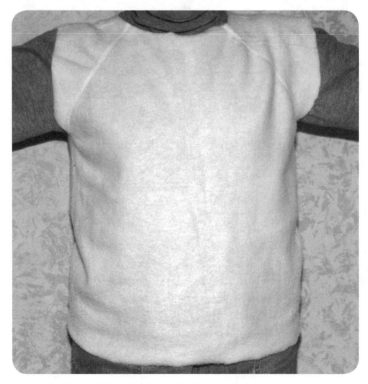

Figure 18.1   Inside-out fleece-lined sweatshirt.

so that the fleece is on the back; that way the organs will stick to the fleece of the vest. (In figure 18.2, the left lung—actually on the right as you face it—is cut from a sleeve.)

3. Use permanent markers to add detail to the organs (figure 18.2).

To Use

While studying body systems, allow one student to wear the vest while peers put the various organs where they belong. You can make several sets so that the whole class can be involved at one time.

Variations

You can also make organs from these materials:

- Felt in different colors for different organs (brown lung in figure 18.2).
- Thin craft foam. Attach the hook portion of hook-and-loop tape to the back (red heart in figure 18.2).
- Foam meat trays (attach the hook portion of the hook-and-loop tape; pink stomach is shown in figure 18.2).

It is preferable for all organs to be made from the same material.

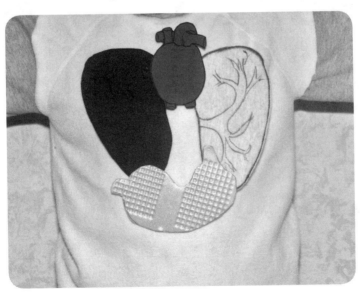

Figure 18.2 Organ vest.

Model Lungs

Models help students see how something works. This model of the lungs does just that.

Materials (Figure 19.1)

- 3 balloons
- Fairly stiff water bottle or soda bottle
- Clay
- 1 or 2 drinking straws
- 2 rubber bands (small)
- Craft knife or scissors

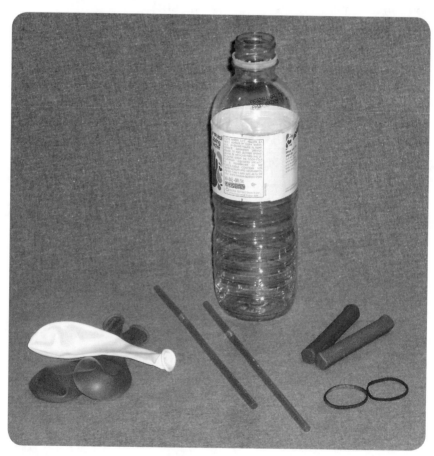

Figure 19.1 Materials for model lungs.

Instructions for Assembling

1. Remove label and lid from bottle. Cut bottom third to half from the bottle. Start the cut with a sharp-pointed craft knife, and use scissors to finish the cut.

2. Cut straws to a length of about 5 inches.

3. With the rubber bands, attach one balloon to one end of each straw. Twist and wrap rubber bands securely, but don't squeeze straws closed (figure 19.2).

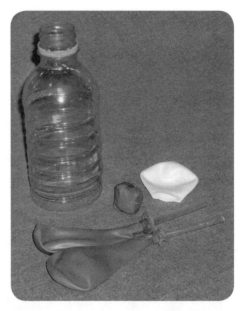

Figure 19.2 Balloons attached to straws.

4. Use clay to make an airtight seal between the open ends of the straws and neck of the bottle. Straws can stick out the top in order to allow the balloon lungs to be located properly in the bottle chest. (They can be trimmed later.) You can use a flat-ended ballpoint to hold the clay in place as you are getting it into the neck of the bottle.

5. Cut off the neck of the third balloon. Use the bottom part to stretch over the open bottom of the bottle to create a diaphragm. (See the bottom in figure 19.3.)

To Use

Demonstrate how the lungs work. Pull downward on the diaphragm (balloon on the bottom of the bottle) and watch the lungs (balloons hanging in the middle of the bottle) inflate. Don't be concerned if the bottom balloon comes off. Simply put it back on.

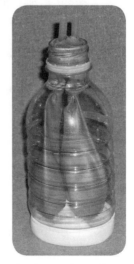

Figure 19.3 Balloon stretches over open bottom of bottle to create a diaphragm.

MyPyramid Pocket Chart

This pyramid hangs on the chalkboard or whiteboard to be used for a variety of activities.

Materials

- White vinyl shower curtain or heavy plastic tablecloth
- Magnets
- Yardstick or long straightedge
- Black permanent marker
- Colored permanent markers (for the colors of MyPyramid)
- Clear plastic tablecloth cover
- Thick craft glue
- Hot-glue gun or clear plastic tape for attaching magnets

Instructions for Assembling

1. Cut plastic sheeting in a large triangular shape or draw a triangle on a rectangle of the plastic sheeting (follow the look of MyPyramid; figure 20.1). You can determine the actual size (approximately 36 inches, or 90 cm, per side).

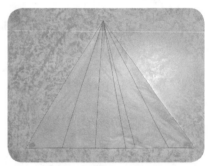

Figure 20.1 Plastic sheeting in the shape of MyPyramid.

2. Draw lines according to the categories of the MyPyramid shape (figure 20.1).

3. Color sections to match the MyPyramid food groups (figure 20.2).

4. Hot-glue several magnets onto the back of the pyramid to allow it to be hung on the chalkboard or whiteboard. Now you can attach magnetic food models onto the MyPyramid.

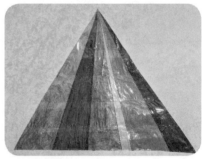

Figure 20.2 Plastic sheeting colored to match MyPyramid.

5. To make a pocket chart, cut 3- to 4-inch-wide strips of the clear plastic that are long enough to go across the pyramid. Use craft glue to secure the strip along most of the lines (to divide the sections), on each outside line, and across the bottom to make pockets over each food group sec-

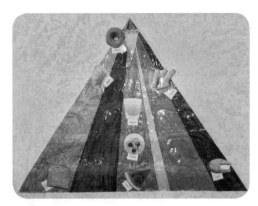

Figure 20.3 Pyramid with clear plastic pockets for pictures of food.

tion. Place several strips up the pyramid so that each section has four or five pockets (figures 20.2 and 20.3).

To Use

1. Use with food pictures cut from magazines (glued to card stock and laminated) or purchased food models (such as from the Dairy Council). You can slip these pictures into the pockets or attach them to the pyramid with magnets glued on the back.

2. With the MyPyramid on the chalkboard or whiteboard, students can do the following:

   • Place food pictures or models onto the pyramid as they learn food groups.

   • Do a relay where students would race to place their foods onto the pyramid into the correct area.

   • Keep a food log for a day and then place their meals on the pyramid in the correct categories.

   • Identify which foods should be eaten in larger or smaller quantities because of the amount of bad fat and simple sugar. For example, if you have whole grains and doughnuts, whole grains would be at the bottom (larger part of the pyramid), and doughnuts would be at the top (smaller part of the pyramid; figure 20.3).

Healthy Placemat

Students can select foods to create a healthy meal.

Materials

- White vinyl shower curtain or heavy plastic tablecloth
- Magnets
- Hot-glue gun or clear plastic tape to attach magnets
- Yardstick or long straightedge
- Colored permanent markers

Instead of purchasing magnets, you can cut advertising magnets into pieces. Since some magnets are not very strong, you may need large pieces of the magnets to hold your items.

Instructions for Assembling

1. Cut plastic sheeting into the shape of a placemat (approximately 12 by 18 inches, or 30 by 45 cm).
2. Draw a large circle for the plate (trace around a dinner plate) and add a smaller circle to represent a glass. Silverware can also be drawn on the placemat (figure 21.1).

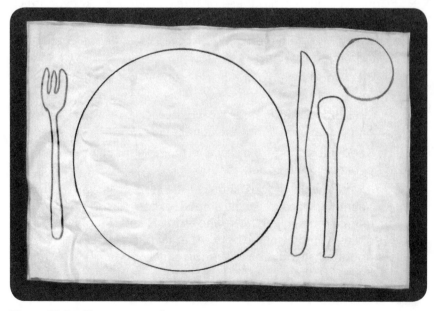

Figure 21.1 Placemat template.

3. Attach magnets to the back. Even with hot glue, putting a piece of clear tape or contact paper over the magnet will help to hold the magnets in place.

To Use

Attach the placemat to the chalkboard or whiteboard. Use with food pictures cut from magazines (glued to card stock and laminated) or purchased food models (such as from the Dairy Council). Glue magnets to the back of the food pictures or models to allow them to be attached to the placemat when it is attached to the chalkboard or whiteboard. (Optional: Use reusable adhesive to attach placemats to wall or foods to placemat.) Students can select foods to create healthy meals (figure 21.2).

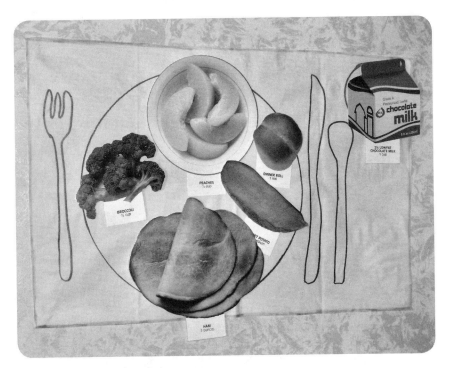

Figure 21.2 Completed placemat.

Simulation of Fat

Use these manipulatives to help students visualize the amount of fat contained in favorite foods.

Materials

- Sheet of wood 1/4 inch thick
- White spray paint
- Yellow spray paint

Instructions for Assembling

1. Cut wood into 1-inch (2.5 cm) squares (at least 15 squares for every group of four or five students; figure 22.1).
2. Lay squares on newspaper to paint. (Make sure it's a well-ventilated area.)
3. Spray with white paint. (White paint has more pigment, which will allow the wood to be covered.) Once they dry, turn them over and repeat.
4. When they're dry, repeat spraying with yellow paint.

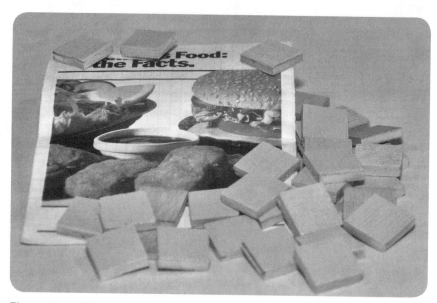

Figure 22.1 Wood cut into 1-inch squares.

To Use

Each fat pat represents 1 teaspoon of fat. Each teaspoon of fat is 4 grams. Give students the nutrition guides from their favorite fast-food restaurants. (These can be printed off the Internet if restaurants don't have them.) Let students select their favorite foods or meals. Figure the number of fat grams in the food or meal, convert that to teaspoons, and stack up the number of fat pats to represent the meal. Repeat the activity, finding healthier alternatives (that is, if most students tend to choose fried and processed foods high in saturated fat, which are the types of food they usually go for!).

Simulation of Sugar

People tend to eat too much sugar. With these manipulatives, students can visualize the amount of sugar contained in their favorite foods.

Materials

- Product labels (with nutrition facts labels) of various cereals, granola bars, and other snacks
- Plastic bags (available in craft stores) approximately 2 by 3 inches (5 by 8 cm)
- Sugar or salt
- Measuring spoons
- Stapler if the bags are not zippable
- Stick-on labels

Instructions for Assembling

1. Select food items that your students eat or recognize.
2. Make a bag of sugar (or salt to represent the sugar) for the amount that is contained in each food (4 grams = 1 teaspoon).
3. Close and seal the bags. (Fold the top down and staple if necessary.)
4. Label the bag with the amount of sugar it contains on one side and the product name on the other side (figure 23.1).

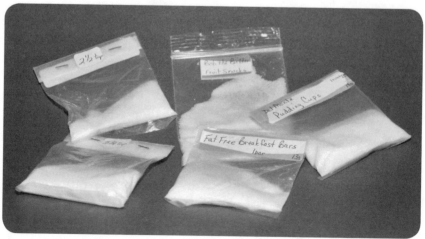

Figure 23.1 Bags of sugar with labels.

To Use

Give each group of students several sugar bags and their correspond-ing food labels (figure 23.2). Let the students guess which bag goes with which food by looking *only* at the side that indicates the amount of sugar in the product. They can check for themselves by flipping over the sugar bags. Discuss any surprises and why foods with raisins or other fruit or dairy products have high sugar content. (Labels don't distinguish between added sugar and natural sugar from the fruit or milk.)

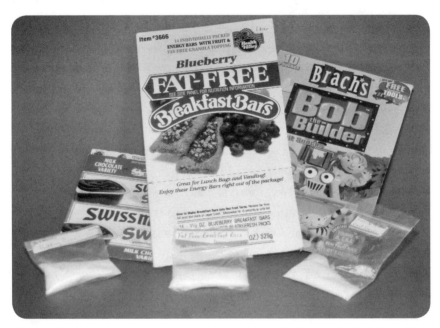

Figure 23.2 By showing only the amount of sugar in the products, let students match up the bags of sugar to the products.

Food Portion Kit

Help your students visualize the size of a portion of food so they can more easily follow the guidance of MyPyramid.

Materials

- File box for 5-by-7-inch cards
- Several of the following: tennis ball, baseball, deck of cards, checkbook, dice, matchbook, nickel, CD case, 3-inch-round mint tin, hockey puck, light bulb shape (mine is a stress ball), computer mouse

Instructions for Assembling

Collect the selected items that represent one portion of food. Store in the file box (figure 24.1).

- Tennis ball: 1 cup cooked rice, medium piece of fruit
- Baseball: 12-ounce potato or 1 cup cold cereal
- Deck of cards (or cassette tape): 3 ounces of meat
- CD case: 1 slice of bread, 1 pancake
- Matchbook: 1 tablespoon oil, salad dressing, or syrup
- Nickel: 2 ounces dry spaghetti (1 cup cooked spaghetti)
- Wood square (or 6 dice): 1 ounce cheese
- Mint tin (or hockey puck): bagel
- Checkbook cover: 3 ounces fish
- Computer mouse: baked potato

To Use

Along with a discussion of how much of each food group should be consumed in a day, these models can help students visualize how much they are actually eating.

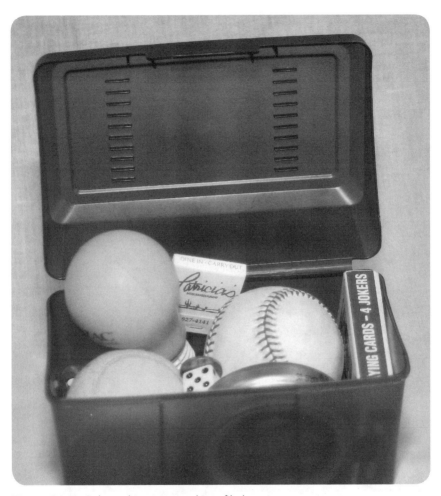

Figure 24.1 Selected items stored in a file box.

Portion Plates

Help your students visualize what food groups and how much of each food group they should eat at a meal.

Materials

- Plastic plates (8 to 10 inches, or 20 to 25 cm, in diameter)
- Markers or plastic knife and fork
- Reusable adhesive
- Paper or food models

Instructions for Assembling

1. Divide plate into half horizontally by either drawing a diagram of a knife or attaching a plastic knife with the reusable adhesive (figure 25.1).

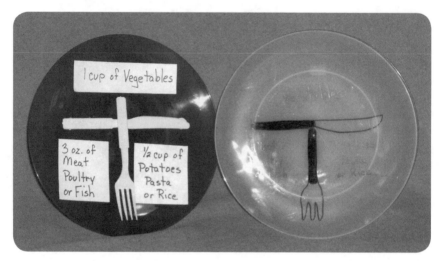

Figure 25.1 Plastic utensils held in place with reusable adhesive work well for dividers.

2. Divide the lower half vertically by either drawing a diagram of a fork or attaching a plastic fork with the reusable adhesive.

3. Using a marker, write portion sizes of foods in correct spaces, or write on paper and attach to areas with the reusable adhesive.

To Use

Students can use the plates to visualize the portions and types of foods in a healthy meal. Or they can place food models into the proper sections of the plate to create healthy meals.

A Pound of Fat

Help your students experience how much a pound of fat weighs.

Materials (Figure 26.1)

- Two 1-inch-thick (2.5 cm) foam strips approximately 4 by 14 inches (10 by 35 cm)
- Alternatives:
  - Felt strips (light yellow to look like fat)
  - Foam drawer liner (yellow), doubled to make it thicker
- 1 pound (.5 kg) of 3-inch (8 cm) nails
- 2-inch-wide (5 cm) masking tape or duct tape
- Hot-glue gun

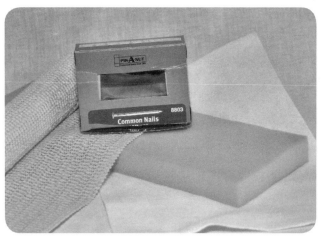

Figure 26.1 Materials for simulating a pound of fat.

Instructions for Assembling

1. Lay out a strip of masking tape or duct tape approximately 15 inches long, sticky side up.

2. Alternate laying the nails head up and head down as close together as possible across the tape. The tape will be used to hold them together side by side (figure 26.2). When you have placed 1 pound of nails on the tape, fold over any extra tape and place another piece of tape over the top to enclose the nails.

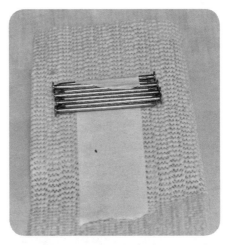

Figure 26.2 Line up nails close together on the tape.

3. Put the strip of nails onto one of the pieces of foam, felt, or drawer liner. Cover with the second piece and hot-glue them together (figure 26.3).

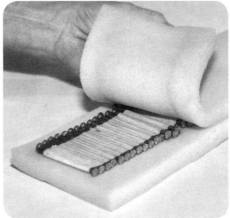

Figure 26.3 Complete the pound of fat by covering the nails with the second piece of foam and hot-gluing the two pieces together.

To Use

Students can hold the "fat" around their bodies to represent how fat accumulates. As they move around, they will experience the feeling of carrying around extra weight.

Fat Vest

Allow students to experience the feeling of carrying around extra weight.

Materials

- Old sweatshirt
- Scissors
- Hot-glue gun (or sewing machine)
- 1-pound (.5 kg) weights: 3-by-6-inch (8 by 15 cm) sleeve created from some tightly woven scrap material (sewn or hot-glued) filled with 1 cup of sand

Instructions for Assembling

1. Cut neckband off the sweatshirt.
2. Cut sleeves off the sweatshirt. Cut wristbands off the sleeves.
3. To create a tube shape, trim excess material from the upper part of each sleeve. Hot-glue the trimmed section of the sleeve shut to form the tube. Hot-glue one end shut (figure 27.1).

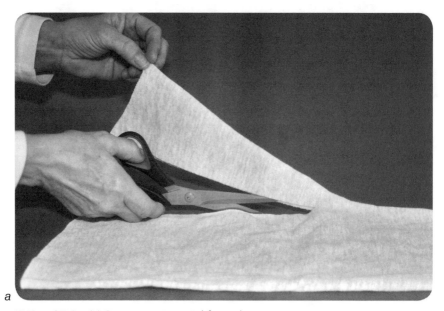

a

Figure 27.1 (a) Cut excess material from sleeve.

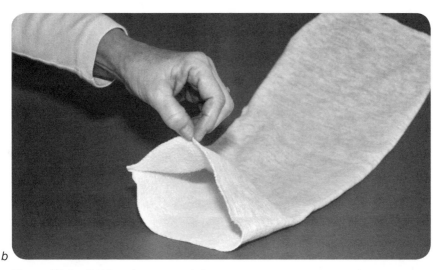

b

Figure 27.1 *(b)* Hot-glue one end shut.

4. Repeat with second sleeve.

5. Attach one tube to the outside front waist of the shirt by hot-gluing it. Attach the other sleeve in the back.

6. Create several 1-pound (.5 kg) weights (depending on how much weight you want students to carry around).

7. Turn the sweatshirt inside out so the tubes are inside the shirt. Slide weights into the tubes to represent the extra weight a person would carry around (figure 27.2).

Figure 27.2 Weights inside the tube, hot-glued to the inside of the sweatshirt.

To Use

Let students try on the vest with various amounts of weight. As they move around, they will experience how it feels to carry around that extra weight.

Dice

Dice can be used for many activities and games. Creating your own allows you the flexibility of sizing and labeling (pictures, words, numbers from 1 to 6 or 1 to 3 twice).

Materials

Option A
- Large sponge (for washing cars)
- Scissors or serrated knife
- Permanent markers

Option B
- Thin craft foam
- Scissors
- Hot-glue gun
- Permanent markers

Option C
- Plastic storage containers (2 for each die)
- Hot-glue gun
- Permanent markers

Instructions for Assembling

1. Option A: Cut sponge into cubes in the desired size for the dice (figure 28.1). Use markers to decorate as you want (figure 28.2).

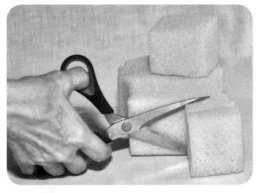
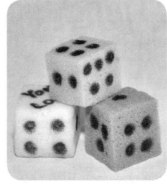

Figure 28.1   Cut large foam into cubes to make large dice (option A).

Figure 28.2   Decorated dice (option A).

2. Option B: Cut six squares in the size you want for the dice. Glue sides together to form a box. Trim if you need to and decorate as you want (figure 28.3).

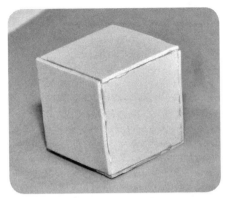

Figure 28.3 Cut thin foam into six squares and glue them together to make a die (option B).

3. Option C: Select containers that will make a box when placed with open ends together. (It does not have to be perfectly square. Having rims around the opening will not affect their rolling ability.) Place objects inside if you want. Hot-glue (or craft-glue) the two containers together and decorate as you want (figure 28.4).

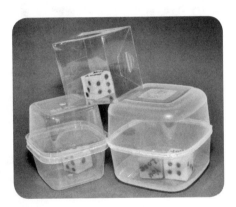

Figure 28.4 Fit plastic containers together to make a box, or double dice (option C).

To Use

These dice can be used in any way you would use regular dice. The double dice (figure 28.4) can have numbers on either the inside or outside die with instructions on the other. For example, the outer die has activities such as jumping jacks, while the inner die or dice have numbers. Students would do the number of jumping jacks shown on the inner dice.

Inexpensive Teaching Props

An ideal place for inexpensive finds is a dollar store. The following are items that can be found in these discount stores. Use your imagination in incorporating them into your existing lessons.

Red Dice

These dice can be used in any way that other dice are used. (These cloth-covered foam dice are approximately 2 inches square.)

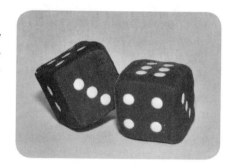

Body Systems Model

These models can be used just as visuals, or students can take them apart as they study the various systems.

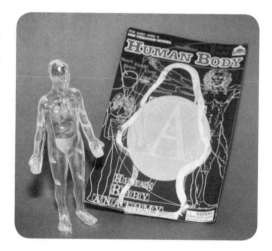

Skeleton Hangman

Let students use this skeleton to play hangman with their spelling words instead of just drawing a stick figure on the board.

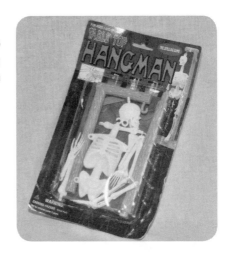

Veggie Magnets

Students can use these magnets with either the MyPyramid pocket chart or placemat.

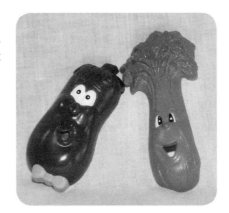

Carrot-Handled Jump Rope

Let students jump rope as they take a break from work. Remind them that carrots make great nutritious snacks.

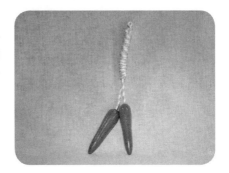

APPENDIX

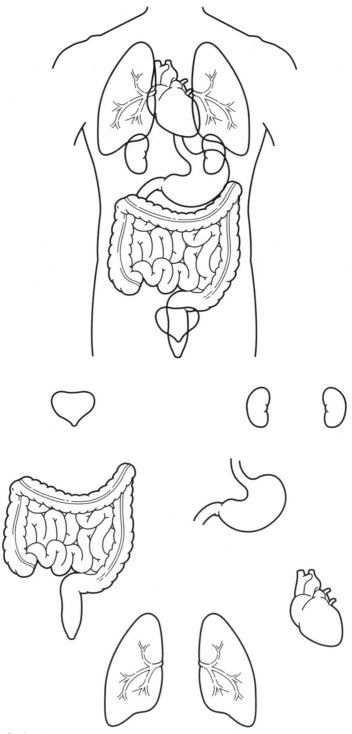

Patterns for body organs.

From M. Grechus, 2010, *Innovative tools for health education: Making inexpensive props, visuals, and manipulatives* (Champaign, IL: Human Kinetics).

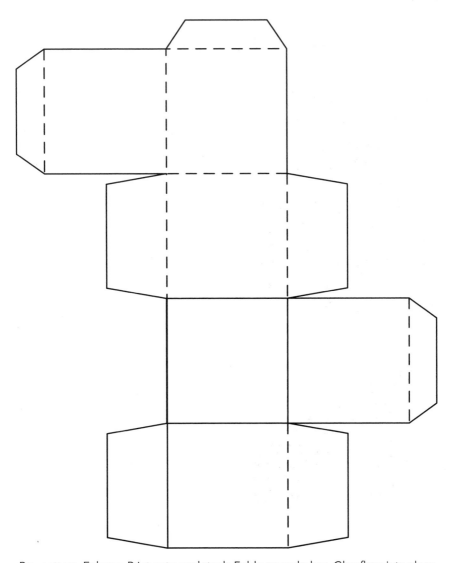

Box pattern. Enlarge. Print onto card stock. Fold across dashes. Glue flaps into place.

From M. Grechus, 2010, *Innovative tools for health education: Making inexpensive props, visuals, and manipulatives* (Champaign, IL: Human Kinetics).

Recipe for Homemade Clay

1 cup boiling water

Food coloring

3 tablespoons salad oil

1/2 cup salt

2 cups flour

1 tablespoon alum (available in the spice section of your grocery store)

Mix together the water, food coloring, and salad oil. Add the dry ingredients. Knead to a workable consistency.

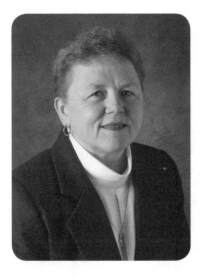

Marilyn Grechus, PhD, is a professor of health education at the University of Central Missouri in Warrensburg, Missouri. She has taught health methods courses since 1992 and has presented on related topics at the state, district, and national levels. She has received two Excellence in Teaching awards, one from the University of Central Missouri and the other from the National Society of Leadership & Success. In 2003 she received the Robert M. Taylor award for professional service from the Missouri Association of Health, Physical Education, Recreation and Dance (MOAHPERD). MOAHPERD also named her University Health Educator of the Year in 2007. In her leisure time she enjoys playing with her grandchildren and doing crafty things.

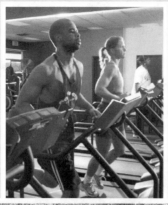
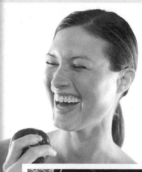
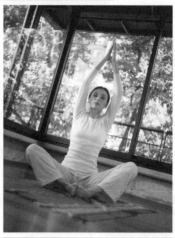
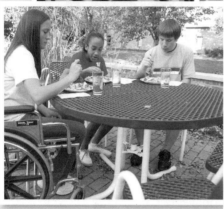

You'll find other outstanding
health education resources at
www.HumanKinetics.com

In the U.S. call 1.800.747.4457
Australia 08 8372 0999
Canada. 1.800.465.7301
Europe . . . . .+44 (0) 113 255 5665
New Zealand 0800 222 062

HUMAN KINETICS
The Information Leader in Physical Activity & Health
P.O. Box 5076 • Champaign, IL 61825-5076